Tiny Hands
that Hold My Heart

words of encouragement for expecting mothers

Tiny Hands
that Hold My Heart

words of encouragement for expecting mothers

Leanne Stevenson

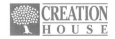

CREATION
HOUSE

Tiny Hands that Hold My Heart by Leanne Stevenson
Published by Creation House Books
A Charisma Media Company
600 Rinehart Road
Lake Mary, Florida 32746
www.strangbookgroup.com

Scripture quotations marked NIV are from the Holy Bible, New International Version of the Bible. Copyright © 1973, 1978, 1984, International Bible Society. Used by permission.

Scripture quotations marked NLT are from the Holy Bible, New Living Translation, copyright © 1996. Used by permission of Tyndale House Publishers, Inc., Wheaton, IL 60189. All rights reserved.

Scripture quotations marked THE MESSAGE are from *The Message: The Bible in Contemporary English*, copyright © 1993, 1994, 1995, 1996, 2000, 2001, 2002. Used by permission of NavPress Publishing Group.

Photos for months 1 and 9 courtesy Photo Researchers, Inc.
Photos for months 2, 3, 4, and 7 courtesy Getty Images.
Photos for months 5 and 8, "Birth Day," "Final Thoughts," courtesy IStockPhoto.com.
Photos for month 6 courtesy Life Issues Institute.

Design Director: Bill Johnson
Cover design by Rachel Lopez

Visit the author's website: www.tinyhandsbook.com

Library of Congress Control Number: 2010940916
International Standard Book Number: 978-1-61638-359-6

First Edition

11 12 13 14 15—9 8 7 6 5 4 3 2 1
Printed in Canada

CONTENTS

INTRODUCTION

ONGRATULATIONS ON YOUR pregnancy! The next nine months will be one of the most exciting journeys of your life. It will be filled with hope, joy, anticipation, and many more emotions too numerous to mention!

Inside these pages you will find a brief description of your baby's development each month. Be in awe of the breathtaking photography that shows what a miraculous creation your little one is and how quickly he or she grows and changes. You will also find specific and relevant scripture that correlates to how your baby is developing.

I hope these verses encourage you and give you a peace that God cherishes the life that is growing within you, and He is watching over your baby's development with the utmost care. So come and take a peek inside to see your baby as God does and may your pregnancy and birth be blessed.

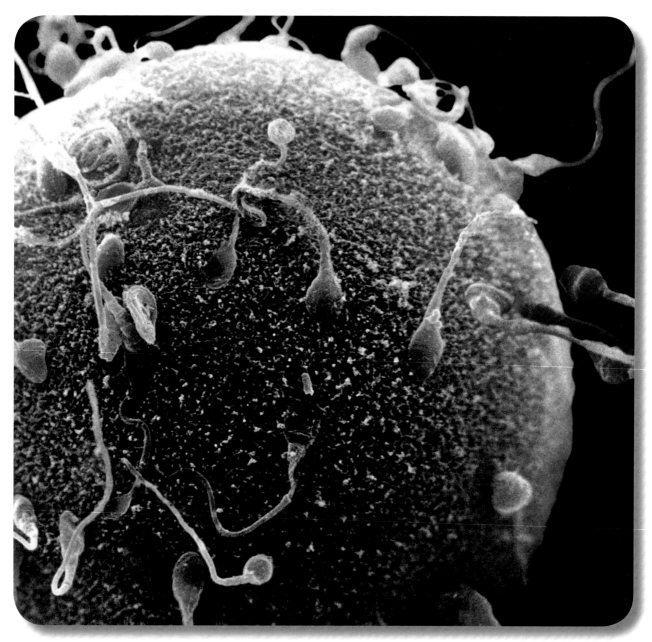

Average weight: .03 ounces

Average length: 1/8 inch

MONTH 1

(Weeks 1–4)

D URING THE FIRST month of pregnancy, fertilization occurs. Cell division and growth begins immediately and rapidly. Your baby begins developing everything needed to survive until birth. The growing cells attach to the uterine wall and start to specialize and group together. By the end of the first month, the placenta, amniotic sac, and amniotic fluid are formed, as well as the beginning of the lungs, brain, and spine. Only eighteen days after conception, your baby has a heart, which is already beating, and you probably do not even know you are pregnant yet.

Before I formed you in the womb I knew you, before you were born I set you apart.

—JEREMIAH 1:5, NIV

You guided my conception and formed me in the womb.

—JOB 10:10, NLT

What an awesome thought—before you even realized you were pregnant, God already knew your baby inside and out. Even now, He already has a purpose, plans, and a direction for your little one. "For I know the plans I have for you," declares the Lord, "plans to prosper you and not to harm you, plans to give you a hope and a future" (Jeremiah 29:11, NIV).

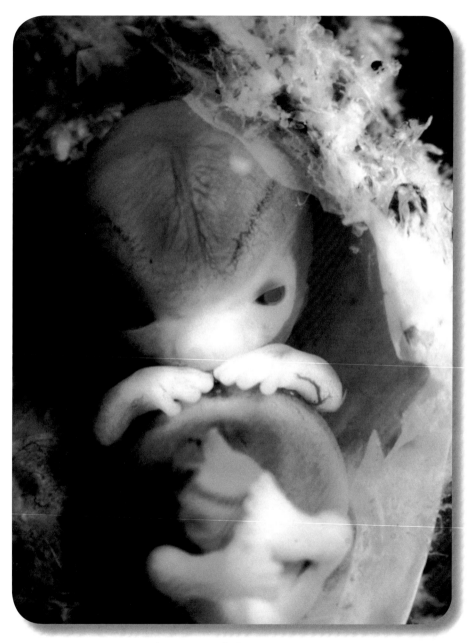

Average weight: .1 ounce
Average length: 1 inch

MONTH 2

(Weeks 5–8)

YOUR BABY CONTINUES to grow and develop. By the end of the second month, all major organs are present. The brain and spine continue to develop. Arm and leg buds form during this month and begin to extend from the body. At the ends are tiny finger and toe buds, each with unique and individual prints. The eyes and ears are beginning to form and tooth buds appear.

> But in fact God has arranged the parts in the body, every one of them, just as he wanted them to be.
> —1 CORINTHIANS 12:18, NIV

> You made all the delicate, inner parts of my body and knit me together in my mother's womb. Thank you for making me so wonderfully complex! Your workmanship is marvelous.
> —PSALM 139:13–14, NLT

God truly did knit us together in a miraculous and marvelous way! Before your baby is even an inch long, all major internal organs are unique and individually formed. The heart is beating and pumping blood. Your baby has fingerprints, toe prints, and DNA that are truly unique and unlike those of anyone else. God loves diversity. When He created your baby, He broke the mold. There will never be, nor has there ever been, another individual that is exactly like your baby. "For we are God's masterpiece…" (Ephesians 2:10, NLT).

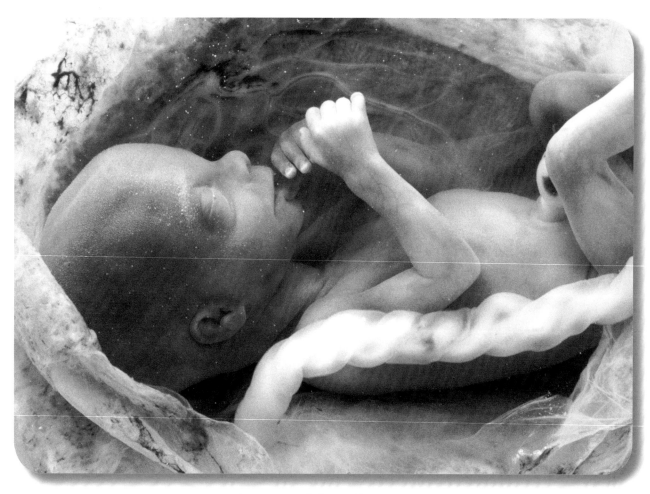

Average weight: 1.7 ounces
Average length: 3.5 inches

MONTH 3

(Weeks 9–12)

B Y THE END of the third month, your baby will be referred to as a fetus and will grow to look more and more like you each and every day. The face has formed, with the eyes, ears, mouth, and nose moving into place. Bones and muscles begin to develop. The brain, nerves, and muscles work together, enabling involuntary movement. Reflexes are present and brain waves can be recorded. Your baby can now squint, swallow, make a fist, and suck his thumb.

> You know me inside and out, you know every bone in my body; you know exactly how I was made, bit by bit, how I was sculpted from nothing into something.
>
> —PSALM 139:15, THE MESSAGE

Human life is truly one of God's greatest miracles. A human being, with all of our intricacies, is miraculously created from two single human cells that combine into one. Life begins with a single, united cell that is smaller than a grain of salt and develops into a person with as many as 50 trillion individual cells, each with a purpose and a job to do.[1] The human body is amazing for what a miracle it is.

> Just as you'll never understand the mystery of life forming in a pregnant woman, So you'll never understand the mystery at work in all that God does.
>
> —ECCLESIASTES 11:5, THE MESSAGE

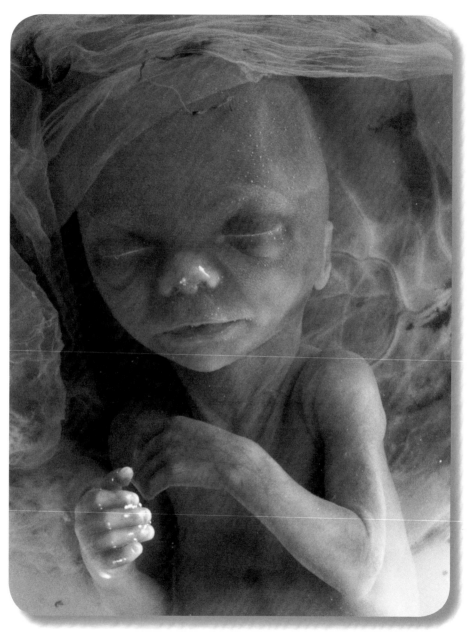

Average weight: 4 ounces
Average length: 6 inches

MONTH 4

(Weeks 13–16)

T HE PLACENTA NOW completely sustains pregnancy. Your baby's ears can detect the beginnings of sound and eyes can detect shades of light. Eyebrows and scalp hair begin to appear. Your baby can produce bile, urine, and insulin from functioning organs. Activity increases in the fetus, which can now kick, grasp, swim, turn, and somersault. However, since your baby is still so small, you will probably not be able to feel it yet. By the end of the fourth month, your baby's gender will be evident with an ultrasound. Will it be a boy or a girl?

> So God created human beings in his own image. In the image of God he created them; male and female he created them.
>
> —GENESIS 1:27, NLT

> For in him we live and move and have our being…We are his offspring.
>
> —ACTS 17:28, NIV

God chose to create your baby because it gives Him pleasure. Although God needs nothing, He loves us and desires to have a relationship with us. Because your baby is created in God's image, he or she will have the ability to know God, love Him, and fellowship with Him. "For you created all things, and they exist because you created what you pleased" (Revelation 4:11, NLT). What a breathtaking thought—the baby growing inside you is pleasing to the one God who created all things!

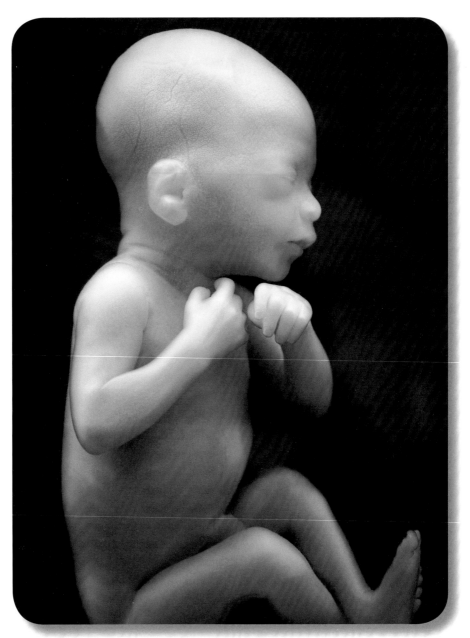

Average weight: 10 ounces
Average length: 10 inches

MONTH 5

(Weeks 17–20)

Y OUR BABY HAS now developed protections from the uterine environment and prepares for the outside world. The developing immune system offers growing protection from infection and illness. A substance is secreted from the oil glands to protect the skin and a soft hair called Lanugo covers the body. A special brown fat is formed to regulate body temperature. Your baby now has vocal cords and can cry. Fetal movement is apparent, and you may soon recognize your baby's waking and sleeping patterns.

Every detail of your body and soul—even the hairs of your head!—is in my care.

—LUKE 21:18, THE MESSAGE

The Lord himself watches over you!

—PSALM 121:5, NLT

Not only has God created your baby with an intricate immune system to protect him against the physical world, but He Himself offers a protection unlike any other. Even the hairs on your baby's head are numbered and in His care. Did you know that the average human has one hundred thousand hair follicles and each of those can produce as many as twenty individual hairs over a lifetime?[1] Isn't it comforting to know that God offers that kind of care and protection for your baby as he grows? "He will cover you with his feathers. He will shelter you with his wings. His faithful promises are your armor and protection" (Psalm 91:4, NLT).

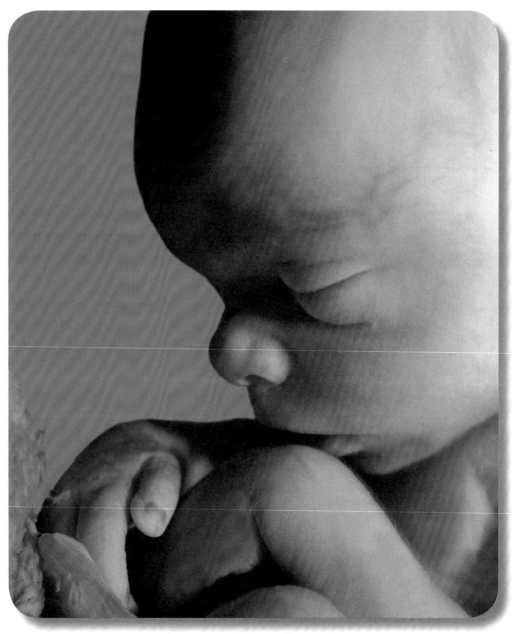

Average weight: 1.5 pounds
Average length: 11.5 inches

MONTH 6

(Weeks 21–24)

DURING THE SIXTH month, circulation to the lungs begins, and your baby will practice breathing. The nervous system is near complete, and the fetus can now feel and respond to pain. The ears have developed enough so your baby can recognize your voice, as well as other familiar sounds outside the womb. Sudden loud noises might even result in a startle reflex. You will also feel plenty of movement this month as your baby is active and still has room to move.

Ears that hear and eyes that see—the Lord has made them both.

—PROVERBS 20:12, NIV

My child, pay attention to what I say. Listen carefully to my words…for they bring life to those who find them, and healing to their whole body.

—PROVERBS 4:20, 22, NLT

Isn't it amazing that when your baby is born, he will recognize your voice and will automatically feel comforted in your presence? He has been listening to you for several months inside the womb. Upon birth, your baby will also be able to hear God's voice and His calling. We have been created to recognize and hear His voice like a sheep recognizes the voice of the shepherd. "My sheep listen to my voice; I know them, and they follow me" (John 10:27, NIV). If your voice as a mother can comfort, console, and reassure your baby, how much more important will the voice of God be as your baby grows!

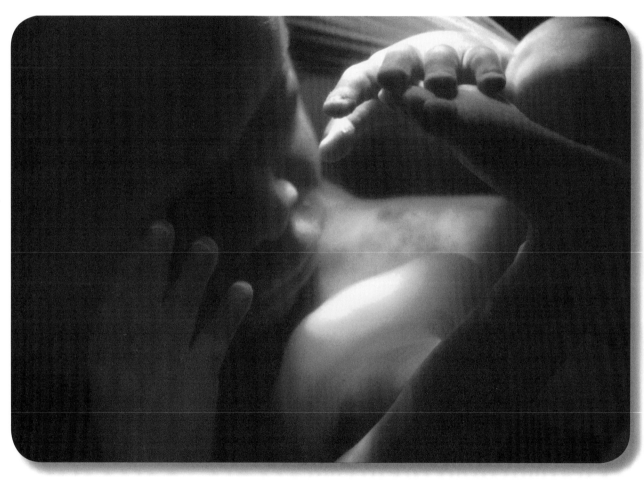

Average weight: 2.5 pounds
Average length: 13.5 inches

MONTH 7

(Weeks 25–28)

Your baby is now growing fast and starting to put on weight. Movement becomes less as space gets tighter and tighter. You might feel a push, a kick, or a wiggle if your little one starts to get uncomfortable. All senses are completely developed—sight, hearing, and taste. Your baby will recognize the music you like, as well as the foods you eat. He is sensitive to bright lights, loud noises, heat, and cold. During this month, there is a tremendous amount of brain and nervous system growth. By the end of the month, your baby should turn head down, preparing for birth.

> From him the whole body, joined and held together by every supporting ligament, grows and builds itself up in love, as each part does its work.
>
> —Ephesians 4:16, NIV

Your baby has been growing and changing from the first day of conception—from one cell to billions of cells. God has been a part of this growth and development from the very beginning. "The Lord called me before my birth; from within the womb he called me by name" (Isaiah 49:1, NLT). He is part of, and will continue to be, part of every aspect of your baby's growth—physical growth, emotional growth, and spiritual growth. "I made you, and I will care for you. I will carry you along and save you" (Isaiah 46:4, NLT).

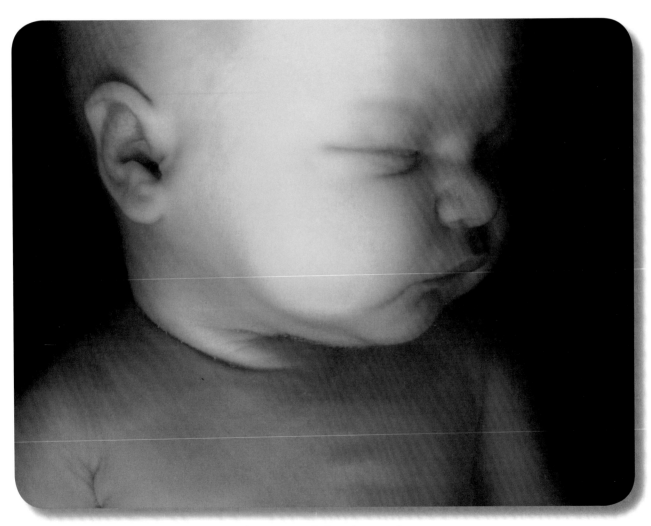

Average weight: 5 pounds
Average length: 15.5 inches

MONTH 8

(Weeks 29–33)

DURING THIS MONTH, your baby will undergo the most rapid overall growth. The baby's weight will double by the end of the month. The lungs will be the last organs to fully develop, but the rest of the body is completely formed. Your baby's eyes can open and shut. Fingernails, toenails, eyelashes, and hair can be quite long by this point. Your baby will to prepare for birth by dropping down into the pelvis. You might begin having contractions during this time and will be anxiously anticipating the birth of your little one!

Like an open book, you watched me grow from conception to birth; all the stages of my life were spread out before you, The days of my life all prepared before I'd even lived one day.
—PSALM 139:16, THE MESSAGE

Yes, you have been with me from birth; from my mother's womb you have cared for me.
—PSALM 71:6, NLT

If you could sum up the physical aspect of pregnancy in a couple of words, they would probably be *growth* and *preparation*. From the first day, your baby has not stopped growing. Growth will continue through the nine months of pregnancy and many years even after birth. The purpose of the initial nine months is solely to prepare your little one for life outside the womb. God has been refining and preparing your baby from the beginning and will continue to be with him throughout his life ahead. "The Lord himself goes before you and will be with you; he will never leave you nor forsake you" (Deuteronomy 31:8, NIV).

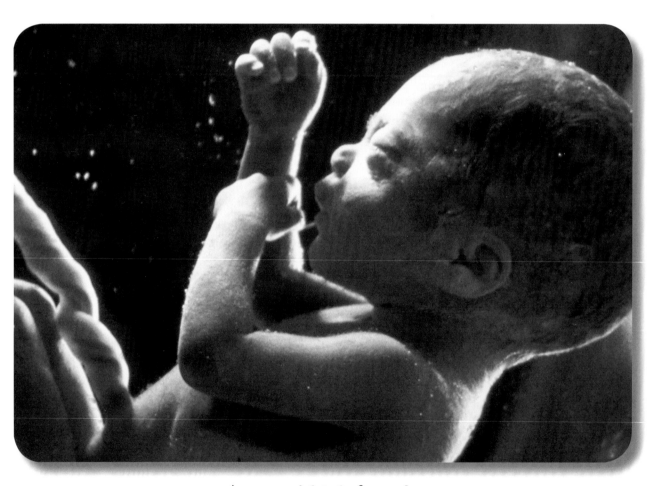

Average weight: 6–8 pounds
Average length: 19–21 inches

MONTH 9

(Weeks 34–40)

Your baby is now ready for the outside world. During this last month, weight gain is the most important part. Your little one should be putting on about eight ounces per week. This added weight will help supply his energy demands during the first few days of life. The protective hair and skin coatings are being shed, and the lungs are developing their final touches. Your baby will be here any day now!

> And I am certain that God, who began the good work within you, will continue his work until it is finally finished.
>
> —Philippians 1:6, NLT

> Yet you brought me safely from my mother's womb.
>
> —Psalm 22:9, NLT

The final weeks have finally arrived. Your baby is fully developed and ready to enter the world. It has been a miraculous, nine-month journey, and God has been with you and your baby every step of the way. Now ahead of you is the awesome and monumental task of delivering your baby. God began the good work of life within you and will now see it through to fruition. You can rely on His strength and comfort during the labor and delivery process. "Look to the Lord and his strength; seek his face always" (Psalm 105:4, NIV).

> I can do everything through him who gives me strength.
>
> —Philippians 4:13, NIV

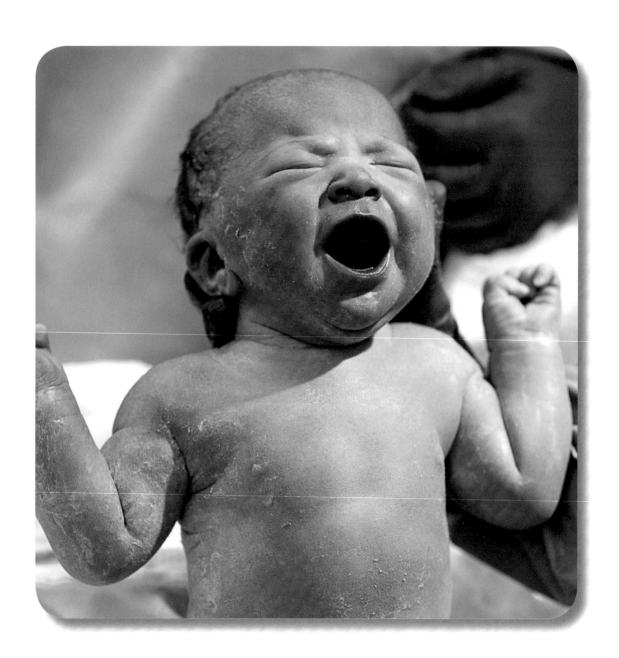

BIRTH DAY

May she who gave you birth, rejoice!
—**Proverbs 23:25**, NIV

OU NOW HAVE a tremendous task to accomplish—the birth of your baby. Near the end of the ninth month, your body will show signs that it is time for your baby to be born. The process that leads to birth is called labor and delivery. There are certain stages that you will progress through, however, each birth process and birth are unique. It will be hard work and at times unpredictable but nonetheless breathtaking and exciting! "When a woman gives birth, she has a hard time, there's no getting around it. But when the baby is born, there is joy in the birth" (John 16:21, THE MESSAGE).

> Children are a gift from the Lord; they are a reward from him.
> —**Psalm 127:3**, NLT

As your baby is placed in your arms, you will feel a joy like no other. All the long months of your pregnancy and the hard work of labor and delivery culminate to a beautiful little baby—God's gift to you. "Every good and perfect gift is from above, coming down from the Father" (James 1:17, NIV).

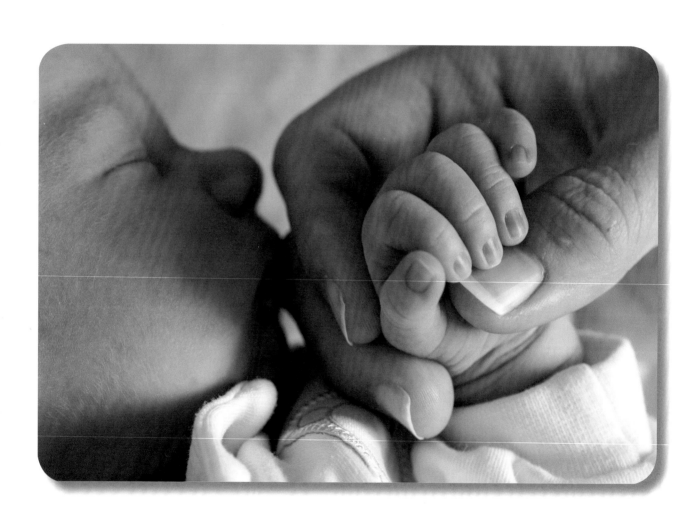

FINAL THOUGHTS

I HOPE YOU HAVE found peace, encouragement, and joy reading these Scripture passages related to your pregnancy. Rest assured, no matter what you face during this pregnancy—the excitement, the anticipation, and the unknown—you have a peace in your spirit knowing God is with you and your baby each and every day.

Each year, it is estimated that nearly 50 percent of all pregnancies among women in the United States are unplanned or unexpected. These women may not rejoice in being pregnant, but will face fear, anxiety, and regret toward the baby growing inside them.

We serve a God who cherishes life and has plans and desires for every single baby, despite the surrounding circumstances. God's Word is powerful, it speaks life, and when it goes out, it does not return empty but accomplishes and achieves its purpose.

A pamphlet-style version of this book has been created with a slightly different Introduction and Finale, written specifically for women facing an unplanned pregnancy. If you know someone who may benefit from the good news and hope within these pages, and would like to send them a copy, please visit our website: www.tinyhandsbook.com.

NOTES

The monthly size and weight estimates were derived from the author's firsthand experience working in and with various pregnancy ministries.

Month 3
1. Found at the website: www.randomfacts.com (accessed October 27, 2010).

Month 5
1. Found at the website: www.randomfacts.com (accessed October 27, 2010).

ABOUT THE AUTHOR

Leanne Stevenson lives in Concord, North Carolina, where she is a wife and mother with three daughters. She is the business owner of BestBabyShower.com and volunteers at her church through the prayer ministries and specialized ministries for adults and children with disabilities. Leanne is a board member of the New Hope Women's Ministry, which helps women who have had abortions find restoration, peace, and healing through the forgiveness of Jesus Christ. This book was birthed through vision, prayer, and God's confirming word from Psalm 45:1.

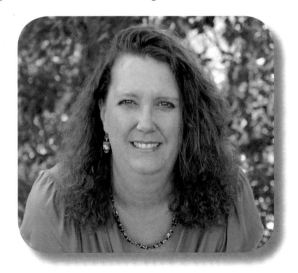

CONTACT THE AUTHOR

Visit the website: www.tinyhandsbook.com
By email: info@tinyhandsbook.com
Or by mail:
Tiny Hands
4525 Motorsports Dr.
Concord, NC 28027